Awakening Series

Breathe

PUBLISHED BY:

Take Abreak

Copyright © 2018Take Abreak

Take Abreak organized a blessing ceremony to fundraise for victims of earthquake. After that event, Take Abreak founded a line group to encourage participants to keep on the meditation shared on the blessing ceremony.

Take Abreak has been sharing a piece of article with group members since then. That's the beginning of this Awakening Series.

1.

Many people breathe shallowly, short and inconstantly.

This breathing style would accumulate pressure in our body and make it uncomfortable.

You can try to adjust it gradually.

Breathe in to your stomach (belly out), then breathe out from your nose slowly (belly in).

Adjust your breathing into the correct abdominal breathing.

It can make your body energy flow free (with other benefits).

You don't have to trust what I said.

Just trust yourself.

Give yourself a chance to do the breathing practice.

2.

Breathe in from your nose to your abdomen, and breathe out from your abdomen to your nose.

This is called abdominal breathing.

It is a natural and comfortable breathing style.

It is a way to transform your body and mind.

It can bring unbelievable changes to you.

We don't have to accept the emotion people bring to us.

When someone offers you a gift, you would not have it if you refuse to accept.

We can decide whether to be happy or unhappy.

3.

When people are in a bad mood, they can not breathe well.

And it is hard to calm down then.

Remember to adjust your breathing.

Breathe in deeply.

Breathe out slowly.

Repeat this a few times.

Breathing correctly can calm your mind and emotion down gradually.

4.

Breathing is the fundamental method.

It is an easy method.

It is the method between arising and ceasing.

Everything is within your inhalation and exhalation.

We are free to make our choices.

5.

Adjust our breathing to abdominal breathing gradually.

Integrate this breathing style into our lives.

Gradually we will discover our brainwaves change.

Our vibration frequencies change as well.

We can get into the state of meditation easier.

We can connect with all things on earth.

We get healthier and healthier.

Generally we think that breathing is no big deal.

Actually it is very important.

We can talk about the benefits of correct breathing way for a few hours.

But you have to experience it for yourself.

6.

Do not cling to the things appeared during
you're in meditation state.

Back to the moderate path.

Clean our inner world constantly.

Bring ourselves back with our breaths.

Every step is a new beginning for us.

7.

The universe is composed of energy, sound and vibration.

When you breathe, you are creating vibration; when you have a thought, you are creating vibration and your awareness is reaching to a different level.

This vibration of breathing then brings your vibrating energy back to you.

8.

We change our brainwave sand nerves with breathing, movements and meditations.

They bring us back to a restful status.

They bring us back to a clear and refreshed mind.

They make us aware of every thought clearly.

They make us remain in the status of samadhi.

9.

Our mind gets steadier and steadier through daily breathing practice.

Quantitative changes would lead to qualitative changes.

We can turn on the key to our bodies, activate the sleeping energy and balance the unbalanced chakras.

We can lead ourselves back to our true selves again.

We will show the feminine qualities which belong to our quiet and gentle inner part.

We will also show our masculine qualities which demonstrate outward strength and braveness.

It can change our magnetic field and rebuild our body and mind.

It can lead us back to the way to abundance.

We will discover that we are living a life of abundance.

Just get rid of the fear in our heart.

Just stay away from all those negative things and people.

Just get close to nature more.

Just listen to good music more.

Just eat clean food.

10.

We do our breathing practice to clean and transform the blocked energy in our sub-consciousness.

We don't have to identify how this happened with our brain.

Our brain would never know.

It is called sub-consciousness because we can not understand it by our brain's functions.

We just need to be aware that this blocked energy is already perceived and coped with.

Then we get over it.

No need to cling to it.

Just focus on breathing with concentration and let the energy flow.

11.

After we have got back to the material world
after experiencing the non-material one, we
would start to yearn for the experience in the
non material density.

We would try hard to go back to it.

But we don't understand.

We are in it now.

We have always been in this non material
density but we think we are not.

We try to escape from the material world
constantly to achieve that kind of status.

But everything is within us, within our
breath.

12.

The law of the universe is you reap what you
sow.

We plant the seeds of kindness, compassion
and willing to help others.

In the world which spins fast nowadays,
soon they will flourish.

We create our own present.

Our present breathing determines our living
quality.

All these secrets await our discovery.

13.

Daily breathing practice improves our concentration and changes our aura.

Our body will then start to heal itself.

There are more benefits.

The spaces we are in will start to resonate with others.

The unconditional healing then starts naturally.

It can not only heal ourselves but others.

14.

Getting into a microcosm through your subtle and long breaths, you can see the congregation and flow of energy.

You will see every face on the street has been changing to your face.

You will see everything presented in the form of lively DNA.

We are all kinds of everything.

We are others.

When you are transforming, do not cling to certain status.

Do not trust what you see from your eyes.

Let all the good and bad flow by.

Just relax and breathe.

Just start to mediate and get into the status of Samadhi.

Just go back to infinity.

There is no such thing called "me".

There is nothing.

But do not afraid of this nothingness.

When you go through all these, you will understand that there is everything within it.

Language can not make you understand tacitly.

I have to repeat again: everything starts with your practice.

15.

If you think that you already achieve the status of thinking nothing, it doesn't mean you have achieved the status of emptiness.

Sometimes it is just because that you haven't started your spiritual practice yet.

You think that you think of nothing, but the truth is that you are just not aware of your chaotic thoughts and your heavy breaths.

You are just led by your emotion or others' speeches.

You can observe your own changes before and after the breathing practices.

16.

Are we living our days or are we pushed forward day by day?

Meditation can make our mind more clear and refreshed.

Abdominal breathing can make us more focused.

17.

Divine wisdom is not that mysterious.

It teaches us the essential elements of life
and the flow of life energy.

Through our abdominal breathing and the
opening of our awareness, our cells will start
to revitalize again.

The method to open our awareness is to do
breathing practice.

18.

Sometimes you try to focus on your breathing, but you see your chaotic thoughts keep flying out.

You tell yourself you should quit all those thoughts.

But the more you push yourself, the harder you can reach a focused meditation.

When you find your mind goes astray, go back to your breath.

At the beginning, you will encounter the process of breathing, going astray, back to breathing, going astray again, and back to your breath once again.

This is a process.

Allow yourself to bring yourself back again and again.

Gradually you can stay in your focused breathing and meditation.

You will feel the change of your body and
mood.

Do trust yourself. Be patient and keep
practicing.

This is like digging a well.

You know there is water beneath.

All you have to do is to dig patiently to
certain depth.

The water you are looking for will pour out
at that point.

19.

How we regard others defines what kind of
people we are at this present.

When we are in a peaceful and loving mind,
we see a beautiful world in front of us.

On the contrary, if we are in a moody mind,
the world reflecting our thoughts and senses
must be unhappy.

All things are constructed with tiny thoughts.

Focus on your breath and do the breathing
practice.

It can lead a path to awareness.

20.

Do the abdominal breathing and be in the
present.

This present!

This present!

This present!

From the point of view of linear time, we
have passed three presents.

And these three presents are all different
ones.

There is no need to go back to the old
present.

The only thing you have to do is to focus on
the present of every second.

You won't go back to the past.

But if we perceive from the point of view
out of time and space, we will understand
that every present appears at the same time.

If you can not realize this now, or if you only understand this with your brain but not your own personal experience, you don't truly understand what I have said.

Be honest to yourself.

Do not deceive yourself.

Take some time everyday.

Stay focused on your breathing.

You will see your own changes.

Disclaimer

The information contained in this book is for general information purposes only. The information is provided by the authors and while we endeavor to keep the information up to date and correct, we make no representations or warranties of any kind, express or implied, about the completeness, accuracy, reliability, suitability or availability with respect to the book or the information, products, services, or related graphics contained in the book for any purpose. Any reliance you place on such information is therefore strictly at your own risk.